Contents

The How-Tos and Wherewithals of Successful Beard Growing

While any gentleman stranded in the wilderness without his straight razor and strop may endeavour to grow a certain sort of facial addendum, it takes the cultured man care, precision and specialist equipment to grow a beard to be proud of. Here are some crucial tips and tools to help you go beard or go home.

BEARD TOOLS

Scissors
A well-styled sir is no one without his silver snippers. The best friend of the fuller-bearded gentleman, it's impossible to go too far wrong with a pair of quality, sharp, straight stainless-steel blades. It is possible to obtain beard scissors for no great expense from high-street shops.

Mini Clippers
Smaller than clippers, but no less useful. If your style demands subtlety, miniclippers are perfect for navigating

your devastating jawline and fixing the fiddlier follicles around the nose and mouth.

Comb

Every beard has big ideas of its own and a comb is essential for encouraging it in the direction you want it to grow. For most, the ideal comb has a handle, finely spaced teeth and is made of strong enough material that it won't break down at the first battle. Some prefer to tame their bearded beast with a brush, taking care not to fluff it by brushing more than once a day, but a comb is essential for cutting and styling.

Beard Oil

As the old beard proverb goes, cleanliness is next to manliness. Although the 'upset porcupine' appearance from a lack of beard styling may have once been fashionable in certain circles, true men know finely groomed face fur is the only way to wear a beard. Beard oil moisturises the face and hair, lending welcome assistance to hair growing in challenging climates and helping to prevent unwelcome afflictions such as beard itch. Smoother and fuller to the touch, your bristles will also be less likely to bristle when it comes to styling.

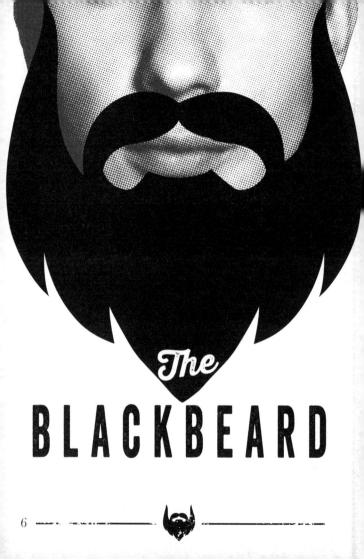

The

BLACKBEARD

EXACTING A REIGN OF
TERROR OVER THE HIGH SEAS,
THIS BEARD IS RECKONED
TO BE ONE OF THE MOST
FRIGHTENING OF ALL TIME.

BRISTLING, PLAITED AND
STUFFED FULL OF SMOKING
FUSES, THE FACIAL FUZZ WAS
SO INFAMOUS THEY NAMED
ITS WEARER AFTER IT.

Grow

DIFFICULTY:

1 Grow your beard and ends of your moustache out until your beard comfortably reaches your chest.

2 During the growing period the beard requires no trimming, but it is necessary to apply beard oil and a comb daily, as the hair needs to be in good enough condition for styling.

3 Divide into four to six large sections and loosely plait, tying off at the ends with a small hairband.

4 Dye your beard black, to match your dark soul. Add beads to your plaits for a dash of piratical swag.

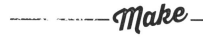

YARN BEARD

DIFFICULTY: 🧔 🧔 🧔
REQUIRED: 1 LARGE BALL OF BLACK YARN,
WHITE PIPE CLEANER, SCISSORS,
PEN, PAPER, FELT

 Draw a Blackbeard template, cutting a space for your mouth and punching a hole either side. Cut the template from felt. Tie ribbon through the holes to fasten round your head when ready.

 Cut the yarn into many separate pieces, each at least a metre long, and combine into at least four bunches.

Loop the sections of yarn in half, divide each bunch into three and plait loosely, tying off at the bottom.

 Glue to the template at the top of the plait – the plaits should cover the entirety of the template and hang off the jaw, ideally to the chest.

The Blackbeard charms and delights when paired with smoking fuses, to give that fresh 'I've just stuck a bottle of rum in my beard and boarded your boat' summer look.

Surprise your friends by accessorising the Blackbeard with a cutlass and musket, bursting into the room and offering them the choice of surrender or death.

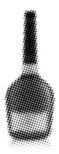

DON'T POINT THAT BEARD AT ME, IT MIGHT GO OFF.

GROUCHO MARX

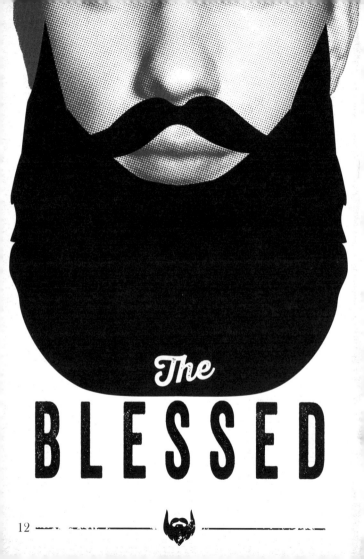

The

BLESSED

BEHOLD THE MAGNIFICENCE AND MIGHT OF THE BIG BUSHY BEARD!

THE PERFECT ATTENTION-GRABBER FOR THOSE UNAFRAID TO ANNOUNCE THEMSELVES. THIS JOLLY GIANT OF A BEARD IS FOR THE BOLD AND EBULLIENT.

Grow

DIFFICULTY: 🧔 🧔 🧔

1 The Blessed, like a fine wine or cheese, is best when it's been matured over many months. The starting point is all-over stubble.

2 As the hair grows, develop the shape. The beard should be trimmed along the sides, but not too closely, maintaining the length at the bottom.

3 The Blessed varies between 1 and 3 inches off the chin; once you have found a length that suits you, trim with scissors to maintain. This beard is too free of spirit to require any grooming products – merely maintain with brushing.

4 Jump on a table to appropriately display your finely furred face to your audience and regale them with acts of derring-do.

BLESSED BEARD

DIFFICULTY: 👹 👹 👹 👹 👹
REQUIRED: FELT, SCISSORS, PINS, NEEDLE,
THREAD, SEWING MACHINE
(OPTIONAL), PEN, PAPER, RIBBON

 Draw a Blessed template on the paper. Ensure the template reaches your ears and has two points that sit either side of your mouth, to fasten the moustache to.

 Pin the templates to the felt and cut around them.

 Sew back stitch around the edges of the felt shapes for a decorative effect. Sew a length of ribbon to the 'sideburns' of the beard shape, long enough to tie around your head.

Pin the moustache to the points of the beard and sew the two shapes together to complete the Blessed.

Charm unsuspecting onlookers by pairing the Blessed with thigh-skimming leather armour and a generous pair of golden wings.

Not only a fascinating facial accoutrement, the Blessed amplifies your voice up to ten times its usual volume, lending your conversation a helpful dash of drama and excitement.

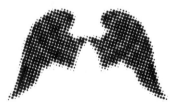

WHEN MAKING A SINCERE VOW, OTTO THE GREAT, HOLY EMPEROR OF ROME, SWORE BY HIS BEARD.

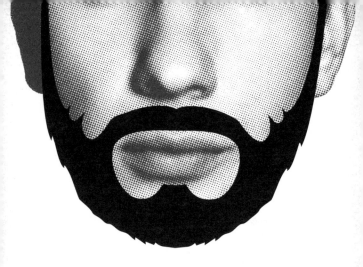

The

EASTWOOD

THIS BEARD IS THE MOST STYLISH ANTI-HERO OF EVERY ROOM. BELONGING TO A GRITTY GOLDEN AGE OF GRIZZLED FACE GROWTH, LOOK IN THE MIRROR AND IT WILL REQUEST YOU

ASK YOURSELF,
'DO I FEEL BEARDY?
WELL, DO YA, PUNK?'

Grow

DIFFICULTY: 🧔 🧔

1 Grow your beard and moustache to about a centimetre in length, or until your face is fully covered with no patches.

2 If you have a high-growing beard line, shave it down to cheekbone height, but do not worry too greatly about neatness.

 Maintain the length with beard clippers.

4 If you are unsure you are wearing the correct length, go for two weeks' hard ridin' on the trail, without shaving. This should create the desired effect.

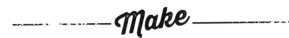

STETSON 'N' BEARD

REQUIRED: FELT, COWBOY HAT, STRING, NEEDLE, THREAD

DIFFICULTY:

 Repeat the steps for felt beard [Blessed], but skip the step for ribbons.

 Don hat, marking on the string where it's level with your ears. Hold beard against face to ensure this is the correct level for you.

 Remove both hat and beard and sew together at marks.

 Stay silent during general conversation, communicating solely through your steely gaze.

The Eastwood is the only facial hair in existence with enough gravitas to allow someone to wear a poncho non-ironically.

If you wish to further style your Eastwood, rub a little dirt into it (dried beans around the mouth optional).

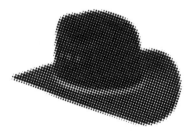

KISSING A MAN WITH A BEARD IS LIKE GOING TO A PICNIC. YOU DON'T MIND GOING THROUGH A LITTLE BUSH TO GET THERE.

MINNIE PEARL

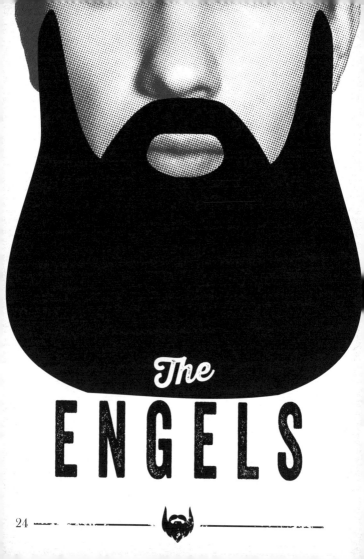

The
ENGELS

SEEN ON FRIEDRICH ENGELS, CO-AUTHOR OF *THE COMMUNIST MANIFESTO*, THE ENGELS ACHIEVES ITS NOTABLE VOLUME BY BEING HEAVY WITH THE WEIGHT OF SOCIAL INJUSTICE.

IT IS OFTEN SEEN ON THE TOWN WITH ITS GOOD FRIEND, THE MARXTACHE.

Grow

DIFFICULTY: 🧔 🧔 🧔

1 Grow your beard out, regularly trimming with scissors to just off the face at the sides, with the length at the chin reaching to around your collarbone.

2 At the same time, grow out your moustache so it reaches your chin at the sides, and trimming to just below your bottom lip at the centre.

3 Although it may be unwieldy, do not part your moustache but maintain it so it covers your mouth.

4 Accept any discomfort this may cause, the road to a utopian moustache is hard and filled with uncomfortable truths.

BEARD NOODLES

DIFFICULTY:

REQUIRED: WET NOODLES, STIR-FRY SAUCE, OIL
PEPPERS, MANGE TOUT, MUSHROOMS

 Heat oil in a pan until lightly smoking, then throw veggies in, stir-frying for 6 minutes.

 Add the noodles, continuing to stir fry for a further 2 minutes.

Add the sauce, simmering for 2 minutes.

 Cover your jaw in noodles – making sure they've cooled – to create a bearded effect, or, alternatively and perhaps more sensibly, eat them.

Comfortably full on noodles, overthrow the capitalist system.

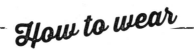

As the Engels obscures most of your face it can be easily used as a disguise with which you may go undercover to observe the unfair treatment of workers.

The style of moustache lying over the mouth filters your voice, lending your words gravitas and making you seem much more profound than you might actually be.

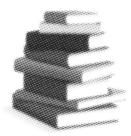

'POGONOPHOBIA' IS THE NAME
FOR THE FEAR OF BEARDS.

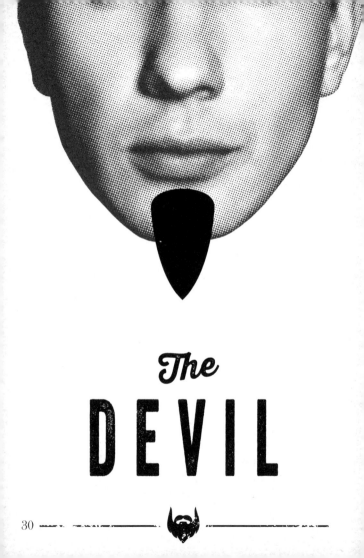

The

DEVIL

MANY WOULD SELL THEIR SOUL TO GET THEIR FACIAL HAIR LOOKING THIS GOOD.

AFTER ALL, A BEAUTIFUL BEARD IS PRICELESS. ALTHOUGH THIS OL' GOATEE IS SURE YOU CAN COME TO SOME ARRANGEMENT...

Grow

DIFFICULTY:

 Keeping your face and neck clean-shaven, grow the hair on your chin to a couple of inches in length.

 For the old-school Devil look, maintain the length with scissors but don't be too careful about precision – you're putting the 'goat' back in goatee.

 For a sleeker, modern look, trim the goatee to a sharp pitchfork point.

 To achieve this, trim the hair through a comb, holding the comb at a 60–70-degree angle. Use a folded mirror to ensure perfect symmetry.

 Offer friends and strangers alike suspiciously good deals.

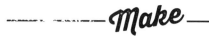

WINE GLASS CHARMS

DIFFICULTY: 😠 😠 😠 😠 😠

REQUIRED: METAL HOOPS, PLIERS, POLYMER
CLAY, TOOTHPICK

 Fashion six beards of any style, no larger than 2 cm, each in a different colour or style, out of the polymer clay.

Slide a toothpick through the sideburns of each beard, and leaving it there, bake in the oven at the temperature recommended on the packet.

When cool, remove the toothpicks. Attach a hoop to each beard through the holes left by the toothpick, then bend the ends of the hoops back so the beards can't slide off. Slip the charms on the stems of the wineglasses.

 Keep the wine flowing at your parties, often asking your guests if you can't tempt them with another glass.

How to wear

From sharp suit to flowing robe, the Devil suits
a wide variety of styles.

If possible, subtly let off smoke bombs
when entering and leaving rooms to create a
suggestion of the hellish dimension about you.

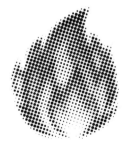

YOU SHALL NOT ROUND OFF THE CORNERS OF YOUR HEADS NOR MAR THE CORNERS OF YOUR BEARD.

LEVITICUS 19:27

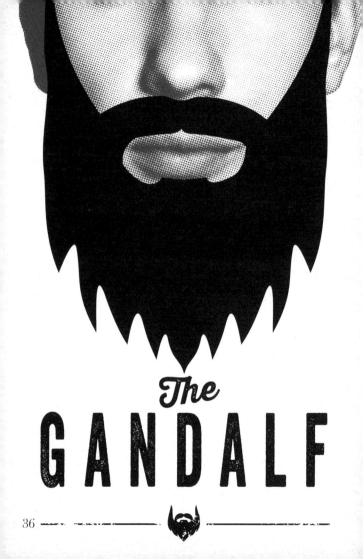

The
GANDALF

FORGED IN BATTLE, POWERED
BY PURE GOOD, THIS
NECK-LENGTH BEARD IS
IDEAL FOR INSPIRING YOUR
COMPANIONS AND STRIKING
FEAR INTO THE HEARTS OF
YOUR MOST EVIL ADVERSARIES.

WARNING: DOES NOT NECESSARILY
GRANT YOU MAGICAL POWERS.

Grow

DIFFICULTY:

 Keeping the moustache trim over your lips, grow your beard until it reaches your collarbone.

 Using a comb to ensure straight edges, trim your beard to a gentle point. The ideal angle to hold the comb at would be around 45 degrees.

 Dye your Gandalf a blinding white.

 As beard hair is naturally course and hair dye takes the moisture out of the hair, the Gandalf will need to be maintained with beard oil.

 Banish bright colours from your wardrobe, wearing only white.

BEARD APRON

DIFFICULTY: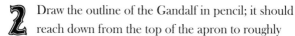

REQUIRED: GREY FABRIC PAINT, THICK PAINTBRUSH, PLAIN APRON, PENCIL

 Ensure your plain apron is a full-body version, which reaches up to your collarbone.

 Draw the outline of the Gandalf in pencil; it should reach down from the top of the apron to roughly chest height.

 In long, downward strokes, paint in the hair. The more visible the distinct strokes are, the more it will look like hair.

 Leave apron to dry.

Don the apron and, holding your staff/wooden spoon aloft, shout 'You shall not stir!'.

How to wear

The Gandalf is to be worn extremely
responsibly – now you appear to be the
pinnacle of wisdom, do not abuse strangers'
sudden love and trust of you.

Don the Gandalf when you wish to add a
dash of excitement to your life. Out of milk?
Quest to the shops. Can't find your keys?
Quest to discover them. Caught in the rain?
Quest for shelter.

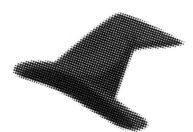

ST WILGEFORTIS WAS A
POPULAR SAINT IN THE
FOURTEENTH CENTURY. SHE
WAS DEPICTED AS A BEARDED
WOMAN, OFTEN WITH A
FIDDLER SAT AT HER FEET, AND
WITH ONE SHOE REMOVED.

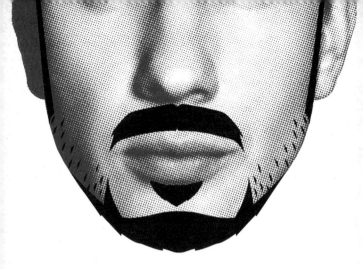

The

GOSLING

HEY GIRL, THIS BEARD MIGHT TECHNICALLY BE CONSIDERED MORE STUBBLE THAN A FULLY- FLEDGED FACE RUG, BUT IT DECLINES TO PUT A LABEL ON SOMETHING AS PRECIOUS AS FACIAL HAIR, AND IS SUPPORTIVE OF WHATEVER YOU CHOOSE TO GROW.

Grow

DIFFICULTY:

 Grow your beard to just past the stubble stage.

 Maintain with clippers, taking care that it looks as if no effort at all has gone into styling your chin chaff.

 If you are over-blessed with even beard growth, use mini clippers to artfully recreate a patchy appearance.

You are now only able to partake of kisses in the pouring rain.

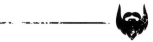

NEON PRINT

DIFFICULTY: 🧔 🧔

REQUIRED: NEON PAINT, BLACK CARD, SPONGE, SHALLOW TRAY, SMALL PHOTO FRAME

 Cut the Gosling out of the sponge.

 Pour the paint into the tray and dip the shaped sponge into it, so one surface is covered but not dripping.

 Print the sponge on the card firmly, ensuring you don't press so hard you blur the edges.

 When the print is dry, frame it. You may need to trim the card in order to fit the frame.

 Have many powerful feelings and attempt to convey them with your eyes alone.

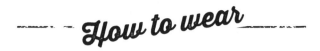

When sporting the Gosling your wardrobe
should walk the paradoxical line of 'modern
retro' and 'new vintage'.

Although your first suspicion may have been
that the quilted silk jacket was a regrettable
impulse buy, the Gosling at last provides an
opportunity to wear it.

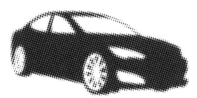

THERE IS ALWAYS A PERIOD WHEN A MAN WITH A BEARD SHAVES IT OFF. THIS PERIOD DOES NOT LAST. HE RETURNS HEADLONG TO HIS BEARD.

JEAN COCTEAU

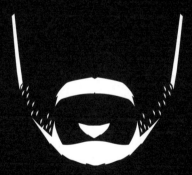

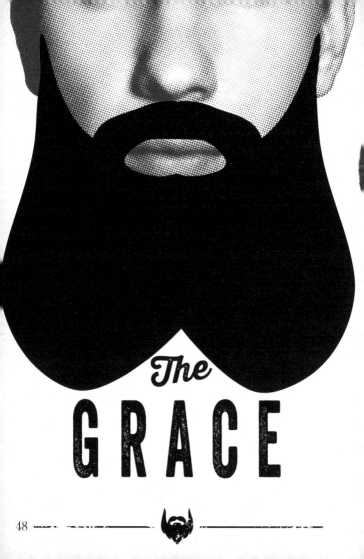

The

GRACE

A RARELY SEEN SPORTS BEARD, CONCEIVED IN THE VICTORIAN ERA BY CRICKETING LEGEND W. G. GRACE. THE GRACE CAN BE SUMMED UP IN THREE PHRASES:

BRILLIANT BOWLER.
BOUNDLESS BATSMAN.
BIG BEARD.

Grow

DIFFICULTY:

1 Grow your beard to the top of your chest, roughly trimming the sides and the moustache with scissors but no comb.

2 Volume is key – this beard is an all-rounder when it comes to size – so maintain with a brush rather than comb.

3 Use beard oil, or lightly wax after you style the hair, to hold the style.

4 Roughly part in the centre and brush outwards to create the broad appearance of two beard flicks.

5 Bring a fierce level of competitiveness to everything you do.

Make

STUD SHIRT

DIFFICULTY:

REQUIRED: SMALL METAL STUDS, FABRIC GLUE, PLAIN T-SHIRT, TOOTHPICK

1 Smooth the shirt on a flat, hard surface. You may need to weigh down the shirt to keep it still – it should be unwrinkled, but not taut.

2 Lay out the studs in the shape of the beard. You can use the studs to create the outline or the full beard, depending on your preference.

3 Carefully, using a toothpick to dab on the glue, stick the studs to the shirt, then wait for them to dry.

4 Due to stalwart uniform rules in cricket, this may be one to wear to your club's soirées rather than matches.

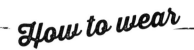

Top your Grace with a jaunty peaked cap in Marylebone Cricket Club stripes.

Regardless of the occasion, wear your best cricketing whites and carry a bat.

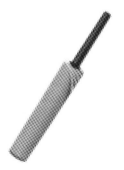

THE WORLD BEARD AND MOUSTACHE CHAMPIONSHIPS IS A BIENNIAL COMPETITION, INCLUDING THE CATEGORY 'FREESTYLE BEARD'. ENTRIES INTO THIS CATEGORY HAVE INCLUDED BEARDS SHAPED AS A REINDEER, LONDON'S TOWER BRIDGE AND BERLIN'S BRANDENBURG GATE.

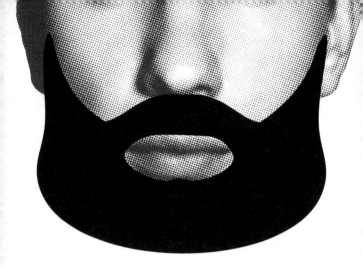

The

HEMINGWAY

ONE PART TESTOSTERONE, TWO PARTS VERMOUTH, THE HEMINGWAY IS PERFECT FOR THE MAN ABOUT THE SAFARI.

THE PAPA OF BEARDS. THIS MUSCULAR MANSCAPE HAS NO TIME FOR LITTLE BOYS WHO CAN ONLY GROW CHIN CHAFF.

Grow

DIFFICULTY:

1 Grow your beard to between 2 and 3 cm in length, keeping the moustache neatly trimmed over the mouth and matching the beard length at the sides.

2 Maintain the length on the cheek with your beard clippers, although you may need to check their shortest setting will keep the hair long enough.

3 Where the beard comes off the face, trim with a comb and scissors, keeping the shape smoothly rounded.

4 Sit down at a typewriter and bleed and/or write.

NAIL ART

DIFFICULTY:

REQUIRED: NAIL UNDERCOAT, COLOURFUL NAIL VARNISH, BLACK NAIL ART PEN, CLEAR NAIL VARNISH

1 Paint your nails with the undercoat and leave to dry.

2 Paint your nails with the colourful nail varnish and leave to dry.

3 Choose two fingers on each hand to be your 'feature nails' and, using the nail art pen, carefully paint beards on.

4 When dry, paint over with clear nail varnish.

5 Write what you know, as long as what you know is hard living, love and loss.

The Hemingway contains so much masculinity
it positively affects objects around it; seize the
opportunity and wear your Hemingway when
drinking cocktails.

Take up a variety of hobbies involving
weaponry and engines.

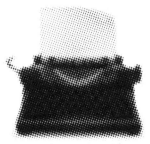

YOU CANNOT GROW A BEARD IN A MOMENT OF PASSION.

G. K. CHESTERTON

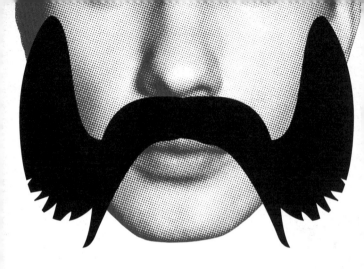

The

LEMMY

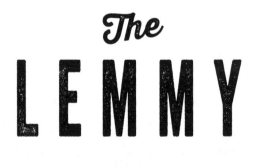

A STYLISH SET OF 'STACHEBURNS THAT ROCK HARD.

THE LEMMY IS A HARD DRINKIN', BIG LOVIN' FACE FLEECE WITH HEAVY METAL CHOPS.

Grow

DIFFICULTY:

1 Grow your beard and moustache about 5 mm in length or until it's full and even.

2 Using clippers, trim all over to a couple of millimetres, so you will be able to clearly see the lines of the style.

3 Use clippers to shave away the hair on your chin and most of your cheeks, leaving sideburns, jawline and moustache fully intact.

4 Create a sharp hairline on your beard using the top of a comb as your straight edge and trimming along it with beard clippers.

5 Add umlauts to any vowels in your name.

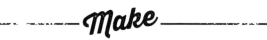

Make

MOSAIC MIRROR

DIFFICULTY: 👤 👤 👤 👤

REQUIRED: BACKING BOARD, STRING, CRAFT KNIFE, REFLECTIVE MOSAIC SQUARES, PEN, PAPER

 Cut a Lemmy template out of paper, lay it over the backing board, and cut round with your craft knife.

 Punch two holes in the tops of the beard for your string to go through.

 Glue the mosaic squares onto the board until there is no blank space, ensuring you don't glue over the holes.

 Thread string through the holes and hang on wall.

 Add a frisson of metal by replacing the string with chains.

How to wear

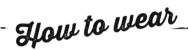

Once you have grown the Lemmy, dye
everything black and add fringing on all items,
including your pants and socks.

Be proud, because you now wear
the ace of beards.

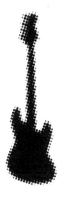

A MALE GOAT SOMETIMES URINATES ON HIS OWN BEARD WHILE RUTTING, IN AN ATTEMPT TO SMELL MORE ATTRACTIVE TO FEMALE GOATS.

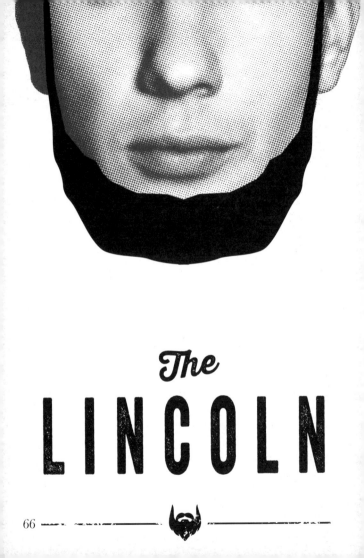

The

LINCOLN

SHORT BUT STIRRING, YOU DON'T NEED TO HAVE STARTED GROWING YOUR FACE FUZZ FOUR SCORE AND SEVEN YEARS AGO TO ACHIEVE THE LINCOLN.

PERFECT FOR WHEN YOU WISH
TO REACH BOTH HEARTS
AND MINDS.

Grow

DIFFICULTY:

 Grow your beard to around 3 cm in length, keeping the moustache area clean-shaven.

 Using clippers, keep the cheeks at a closer shave, barely a couple of millimetres.

 Use a comb and scissors to trim, keeping the hair coming off the jaw and under the neck at a flat, even length, in a roughly square shape.

 Take your Lincoln out on the town, but avoid theatres.

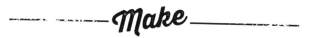

Make

BEARD BUNTING

DIFFICULTY: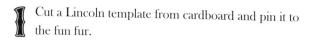

REQUIRED: FUN FUR, CARDBOARD, NEEDLE, THREAD, BIAS BINDING TAPE, PINKING SHEARS

1 Cut a Lincoln template from cardboard and pin it to the fun fur.

2 Using pinking shears to avoid fraying, cut out the beard. Repeat until you are satisfied you have enough to create your bunting.

3 Sew the beards to the binding tape using a running stitch, ensuring they are evenly spaced along the tape.

4 Hang the bunting about the house in order to celebrate your beard presidency.

Seize any opportunity to display your oratory
prowess when sporting the Lincoln.

So widely admired is the Lincoln that it features
on currency and postage stamps, so people may
carry the fine beard wherever they go.

THE WORLD RECORD FOR THE LONGEST BEARD HELD BY A LIVING MALE IS 7 FT 9 IN. AND BELONGS TO SARWAN SINGH OF CANADA.

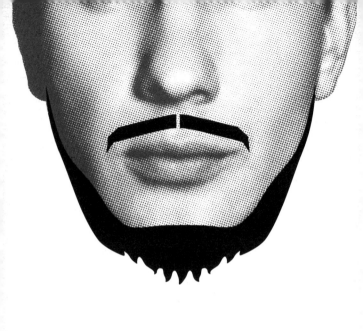

The

MARLEY

 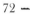

BOB MARLEY WAS A RADICAL THINKER AND MUSIC ICON, PIONEERING THE BURGEONING REGGAE GENRE

AND THE UNDER-LOVED CHINSTRAP BEARD.

DIFFICULTY:

1 Keep your face and top lip clean-shaven, solely growing the hair on your neck to a couple of inches in length.

2 Trim with scissors only to maintain the length and a roughly rounded shape; exactness is not a priority.

3 Bewail your most famous hit 'No Chinstrap, No Cry'.

Make

CRESS BEARD

DIFFICULTY: 🧔 🧔 🧔

REQUIRED: CRESS SEEDS, PLASTIC CONTAINER, WATERING CAN, KITCHEN ROLL OR COTTON WOOL

 Line your container with either kitchen roll or cotton wool and water until soaked.

 Sprinkle the cress seeds in the shape of the Marley, keeping the seeds close together for the best effect.

 Place in the sunshine and water regularly so the lining is kept wet.

 Harvest in a week, once the seeds are grown to roughly 5 cm.

 Eat in a delicious salad, because a man with a Marley loves his green.

In order to make your chinstrap passable,
endeavour to be one of the coolest people
to have lived.

Now that you sport the Marley, don't be
surprised when you find your image gazing
back from every university freshman's
wall and T-shirt.

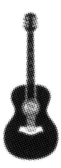

SEIZE OPPORTUNITY BY THE BEARD, FOR IT IS BALD BEHIND.

BULGARIAN PROVERB

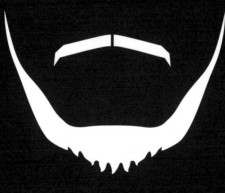

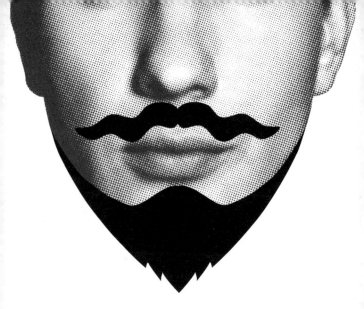

The

SHAKESPEARE

WHAT'S IN A BEARD? A FACE RUG BY ANY OTHER NAME WOULD LOOK AS FINE.

AS CAREFULLY PRUNED AND POINTED AS HIS PROSE, THE SHAKESPEARE IS THE MOST ACCLAIMED LITERARY BEARD.

Grow

DIFFICULTY: ❤ ❤ ❤

1 Grow your moustache and beard to roughly 3 cm in length, or until the beard is comfortably off the face.

2 Do not trim your tache but rather part it in the middle and smooth out into little flicks, fixing with wax.

3 Use a comb and scissors to trim the hair off the face, following the jawline in a rounded shape, but coming to a point at the centre of the chin.

4 Write a sonnet to your newly beautiful beard.

BEARD CUSHION

DIFFICULTY:

REQUIRED: PLAIN CUSHION COVER, FUR MATERIAL, SCISSORS, FABRIC GLUE, PEN, PAPER

1 Create a Shakespeare template from paper, then cut the beard shape out of the fabric fur.

2 Make sure your cushion cover is empty and flat on a hard surface. Apply the fabric glue evenly to the non-furry side.

3 Smooth the beard onto the centre of the cushion and leave to dry.

4 Use the cushion to ease your bony starving-artist backside on the long nights you spend scribbling genius verse.

The Shakespeare has been known to cause unusual side effects, including speaking in blank verse, 'monologueing' and, most unusually, talking eloquently to the person you are attracted to.

Traditionally paired with hose and pantaloons, this is thankfully no longer mandatory and indeed only for the supremely confident.

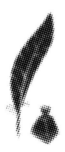

HE THAT HATH A BEARD IS MORE THAN A YOUTH, AND HE THAT HATH NO BEARD IS LESS THAN A MAN.

WILLIAM SHAKESPEARE

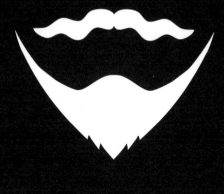

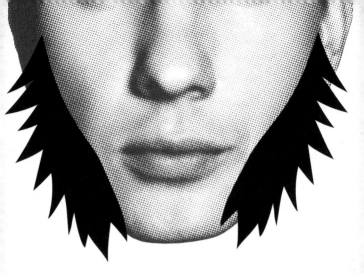

The

WOLVERINE

THE WOLVERINE IS IDEAL FOR ANY BEARD LOVER LOOKING TO SPORT THAT 'I'M A BARELY TAMED ANIMAL' LOOK.

THESE OVERSIZED CHOPS SHOULD REACH YOUR RUGGED JAWLINE AND BRISTLE WITH ANGST AND FURY. GRRR!

Grow

DIFFICULTY:

1 Keeping your top lip, neck and chin clean-shaven, grow your sideburns down until they reach your mouth.

2 Maintain growth until your chops reach an inch.

3 Tease with wax so the hair sticks out with the appearance of controlled tendrils rather than untamed bush.

4 Snip your cigar with your claws, then light it on something conveniently burning close by.

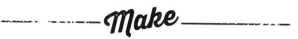

BEARD CAKE

DIFFICULTY:

REQUIRED: CLASSIC VICTORIA SPONGE CAKE, FONDANT ICING, CHOCOLATE FLAKES, BUTTERCREAM ICING, SMARTIES, WRITING ICING

1 Ice the cake with the fondant icing, smoothing over the top to ensure there are no bumps on the cake 'face'.

2 Place two smarties on the face for eyes and use the writing icing to mark on the nose and eyebrows.

3 Using a knife, spread a thin layer of buttercream icing in the shape of the beard. Cover with crumbled chocolate flake to create the hair. If the beard is extra-long it can extend down the sides of the cake.

4 Be a gracious host by slicing the cake with your claws.

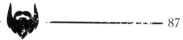

The Wolverine is tough – this distinctive style can survive almost any attack, including the devastating 'change in fashionable opinion'.

You may find your recovery rate from shaving cuts rapidly improves with the Wolverine. This is excellent news – no need to wear uncouth scraps of toilet roll on your face to stem bleeding.

CHINS WITHOUT BEARDS DESERVE NO HONOUR.

SPANISH PROVERB

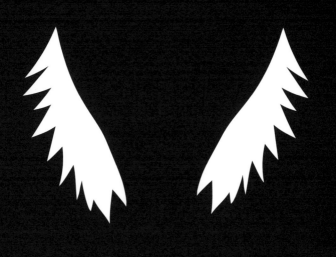

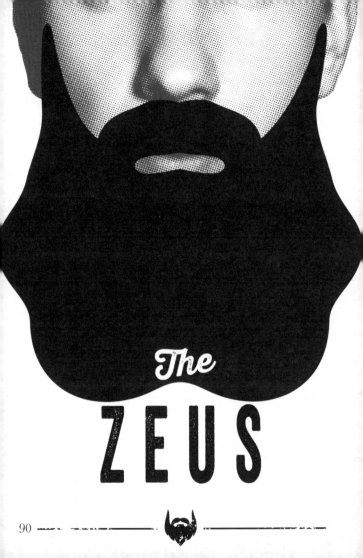

The
ZEUS

MADE OF EQUAL PARTS THUNDER AND LIGHTNING, THE ZEUS IS A CLASSIC.

THE ORIGINAL SILVER FOX.
THIS RIOT OF CURLS AND
LUST IS A GOD AMONG BEARDS.

Grow

DIFFICULTY:

1 Grow your beard until several inches in length, trimming the moustache off the lip.

2 If your beard hair falls into natural ringlets, fortuitous news! You may advance to the last step.

3 Maintain hair condition with beard oil – the Zeus must be capable of holding a shape.

4 Using thin hair rollers or narrow curling tongs, curl your beard all over.

5 Be vigilant for an increased inclination to fall for uninterested princesses.

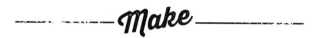
FAKE BEARD

DIFFICULTY: 🧔 🧔 🧔 🧔

REQUIRED: GREY FLEECE FABRIC, SCISSORS, GLUE, PEN, PAPER, RIBBON

 Create a paper template for your Zeus and use this to cut out your beard base using the fleece.

Cut the remaining fleece lengthwise, into 30-cm-long, 1-cm-wide strips. Pull taut and hold for a few seconds and release to create the curls.

 Stick the curls along the beard section, covering the moustache section with uncurled strips of fleece.

 Cut a hole either side of the fleece and attach ribbons that are long enough tie around your head.

 Smite somebody, if it's that sort of day.

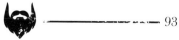

How to wear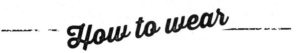

Be extremely cautious who you allow to view
your Zeus – seeing the beard in its natural form
can be too much for mortal eyes.